MEDICAL PRACTICE MANAGEMENT

Body of Knowledge Review

Second Edition

VOLUME 6

Patient Care Systems

Medical Group Management Association
102 Inverness Terrace East
Englewood, CO 80112-5306
877.275.6462
mgma.com

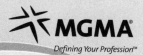

Medical Group Management Association® (MGMA®) publications are intended to provide current and accurate information and are designed to assist readers in becoming more familiar with the subject matter covered. Such publications are distributed with the understanding that MGMA does not render any legal, accounting, or other professional advice that may be construed as specifically applicable to an individual situation. No representations or warranties are made concerning the application of legal or other principles discussed by the authors to any specific factual situation, nor is any prediction made concerning how any particular judge, government official, or other person will interpret or apply such principles. Specific factual situations should be discussed with professional advisors.

PRODUCTION CREDITS
Publisher: Marilee E. Aust
Composition: Glacier Publishing Services, Inc.
Cover Design: Ian Serff, Serff Creative Group, Inc.

LIBRARY OF CONGRESS CATALOGING-IN-PUBLICATION DATA

Patient care systems.
    p. ; cm. — (Medical practice management body of knowledge review (2nd ed.) ; v. 6)
  Includes bibliographical references and index.
  ISBN 978-1-56829-335-6
1. Medicine—Practice. 2. Medical offices—Management. 3. Medical appointments and schedules. I. Medical Group Management Association. II. Series.
  [DNLM: 1. Patient Care Management—organization & administration. 2. Clinical Competence. 3. Health Knowledge, Attitudes, Practice. 4. Patient Satisfaction. 5. Referral and Consultation. 6. Treatment Outcome. W 84.7 P29755 2008]
  R728.P385 2008
  610.68—dc22

                                                            2008044476

Printed in the United States of America
10 9 8 7 6 5 4 3 2 1

Dedication

To our colleagues in the profession
of medical practice management
and to the groups that support us
in our efforts to serve our profession.

Body of Knowledge Review Series — Second Edition

Contents

Preface

TO SUCCEED AND FLOURISH in the day-to-day work environment of managing a medical practice, it is important that the successful administrator master and become adept at utilizing basic and advanced Patient Care Systems skills.

The Patient Care Systems domain within the *Medical Practice Management Body of Knowledge (BOK), second edition,* presents the basic building blocks needed to efficiently and effectively manage the day-to-day operations of a medical group practice, regardless of its legal or political structure. Included within the general competency of critical thinking skills, the Patient Care Systems domain requires an in-depth understanding of the other competencies for the effective management of a group practice.

When faced with the task of assuming the leadership of a medical practice, the effective medical practice executive should properly utilize the basic tools of Patient Care Systems and its patients directly to properly evaluate the issues affecting the organization. Through the proper application of these tools, the administrator will be able to prepare and implement the steps needed to place the organization on a firm footing for survival and growth. Examples of the organizational effects that result when these tools are put to proper use can be seen in many organizations and real life experiences.

Knowledge of the tools within the Patient Care Systems domain and the way they interact with the other domains within the BOK affords the health care administrator the ability to provide the direction and leadership needed by his or her organization. These same tools are utilized in the day-to-day operation of a practice and assist the administrator in ensuring the continued growth and development of the organization.

Body of Knowledge Review Series Contributors

Geraldine Amori, PhD, ARM, CPHRM
Douglas G. Anderson, FACMPE
James A. Barnes, MBA
Fred Beck, JD
Jerry D. Callahan Jr., CPA
Anthony J. DiPiazza, CPA
David N. Gans, MSHA, FACMPE
Robert L. Garrie, MPA, RHIA
Edward Gulko, MBA, FACMPE, FACHE, LNHA
Kenneth T. Hertz, CMPE
Steven M. Hudson, CFP, CFS, CRPC
Jerry Lagle, MBA, CPA, FACMPE
Michael Landers
Gary Lewins, FACMPE, CPA, FHFMA
Ken Mace, MA, CMPE
Jeffrey Milburn, MBA, CMPE
Michael A. O'Connell, MHA, FACMPE, CHE
Dawn M. Oetjen, PhD, MHA
Reid M. Oetjen, PhD, MSHSA
Pamela E. Paustian, MSM, RHIA
David Peterson, MBA, FACMPE
Lisa H. Schneck, MSJ
Frederic R. Simmons Jr., CPA
Thomas E. Sisson, CPA
Donna J. Slovensky, PhD, RHIA, FAHIMA
Jerry M. Trimm, PhD, FHIMSS
Stephen L. Wagner, PhD, FACMPE
Lee Ann H. Webster, MA, CPA, FACMPE
Susan Wendling-Aloi, MPA, FACMPE
Warren C. White Jr., FACMPE
Lawrence Wolper, MBA, FACMPE, CMC
Lorraine C. Woods, FACMPE
James R. Wurts, FACMPE

Learning Objectives

AFTER READING THIS VOLUME, the medical practice executive will be able to accomplish the following tasks:

- Establish and monitor business processes to ensure effective and efficient clinical operations;

- Provide relevant and accurate resources to enhance patients' knowledge, understanding, and participation in their medical care;

- Develop and implement a referral management process;

- Design efficient patient flow patterns to maximize physician schedules;

- Maximize the patient's experience;

- Manage front-office operations to maximize patient satisfaction, collection of payments, and customer service efforts; and

- Implement a plan to control pharmaceutical supplies.

Read It and Weep: "Hidden Epidemic" of Health Illiteracy Hurts Treatment Outcomes[1]

IF MR. A REFUSES TO EXERCISE and lay off the sweets, you'd expect that he won't gain control over his Type II diabetes. If Ms. B constantly forgets to take her blood pressure medication, it's no surprise that her hypertension persists. But did it ever occur to her doctor that if Ms. C is still struggling with asthma, it may be because she can't read the care instructions he gave her?

◾ Poor Health Literacy: A Predictor of Poor Health Outcomes

"Limited literacy skill is one of the strongest predictors for poor health outcomes," says Suzanne Graham, PhD, RN, director of patient safety, California regions, Kaiser Permanente, Oakland, Calif. When patients cannot read and understand basic health information, their ability to comply with treatment regimens inevitably declines. And the extent of illiteracy affects about one in three people in the United States.[2] Approximately 44 million

Americans – 21 percent to 23 percent – are functionally illiterate; about 50 million more are marginally illiterate.[3] Graham calls health illiteracy a "hidden epidemic."

Adults with low health literacy:

- Are often less likely to comply with prescribed treatment and self-care regimens;[4]
- Make more medication or treatment errors;[5]
- Fail to seek preventive care;[6]
- Are at higher risk for hospitalization than people with adequate literacy skills;[7]
- Remain in the hospital nearly two days longer;[8] and
- Lack skills to negotiate the health care system.[9]

Limited health literacy is expensive, she notes. Research shows that it costs the health care system as much as $73 billion annually.[10]

◼ How Do You Know?

Patients unable to read and write rarely declare themselves. Shame leads them to conceal the deficit. Low-literacy patients can be well-spoken and articulate, but certain behaviors provide clues. A practice administrator must remind physicians to be on the alert for patients who may:

- Seek care only when an illness is advanced;
- Frequently miss appointments;
- Skip tests and referrals;
- Fail to comply with treatment plans; or
- Say "I'll read it later," "I don't have my glasses," "Let me take it home to discuss with my spouse [children, etc.]" when presented with self-care material.

Low health literacy equates to problems with:

- Medicines;
- Appointment slips;

- Informed consent;
- Self-care instructions; and
- Health education materials.

You can't identify a low-literacy patient just by looking, Graham warns. "And it's so important not to embarrass the patient."

◢ A Risk to Patient Safety

Patients with low health literacy are at greater risk for injury and medical errors. Unable to read medication labels, they may take the wrong dose. They may take the wrong drug altogether, if prescribed more than one medication. Low-literacy patients often recognize their prescriptions by the appearance of the label – and many packages look similar, Graham notes.

Who is most likely to have low literacy? Those:

- From other countries, now learning English;
- Who did not complete high school;
- Aged 65 and older;
- With physical, mental or health conditions that keep them from participating fully in work, school or other activities; or
- With visual difficulties.[11]

Low-literacy patients may try to memorize spoken instructions. Forgetting or misunderstanding can lead to an accident.

While the average reading level of U.S. adults is between the eighth and ninth grade,[12] "most information given to patients is at the high school level or above," Graham says.

This means that your practice may provide patients material far beyond their reading comprehension. "It's very hard to get complex medical information to a level that most patients can understand, but we have to try," Graham emphasizes.

◼ What Can We Do?

Working with your clinical and administrative staff, create a shame-free environment so patients don't feel embarrassed about low literacy. Promote assessment techniques to identify these patients. Create patient-friendly written materials and encourage clinicians and staff to improve their communications with patients.

Graham says that caregivers should teach patients to ask three questions:

1. What is my main problem?
2. What do I need to do for my main problem?
3. Why is it important for me to do this?

Encourage your practice's caregivers to use "teach-back": have them ask patients to describe their understanding of what's been discussed and recommended. Clinicians should check the family's understanding of these points, as well.

Teach-back is especially important when clinicians:

- Prescribe new medications;
- Explain new diagnoses;
- Give home-care instructions; and
- Demonstrate the use of medical devices.

Understanding is a two-way street. There's a big difference between a clinician asking, "Do you understand what we've talked about?" and "Tell me what we've talked about." Is your practice alert to helping low-literacy patients?

Current Patient Care Systems Issues

WHEN LOOKING at the Patient Care Systems domain from a broad perspective, it is clear that this domain is in a state of change. It is apparent that the domain is in a state of evolution as it attempts to maintain balance while also changing to meet the demands and expectations of the individual stakeholders as well as society as a whole. The practice administrator should take the time to identify and understand the specific pressures of operations as well as those issues that are core within other domains but also affect this domain.

Numerous internal and external pressures affect the patient/clinical side of practice management. These pressures include, but are not limited to:

1. Controlling pharmaceuticals;
2. Patient flow;
3. Patient education and expectations;
4. Staff and physician expectations; and
5. Community expectations/public relations.

Knowledge Needs

TO PROPERLY AND EFFECTIVELY RESPOND to the ongoing internal and external forces on both the practice and business of medicine, the practice executive should be well grounded in the fundamentals of day-to-day operations and the methodologies needed to maintain and improve the processes that affect organizations during these ever-evolving times. Expertise in these fundamental Patient Care Systems skills is the ultimate goal.

Several of the key skills include the ability to ensure effective and efficient clinical operations; provide relevant patient educational systems; enact efficient patient flow patterns; and maximize patient satisfaction. Finally, the medical practice executive needs to know how the various parts of the operation fit together and how they complement and support each other.

Patient Care Systems includes seven distinct tasks, as identified in this volume. Each task is interconnected with the others through a few strong identifiable threads, namely these two:

1. Analyzing how a patient moves through the practice; and

2. Managing the billing, collections, and pharmaceuticals.

Chapter 1   # Ensuring Effective and Efficient Clinical Operations[13]

GOOD COMMUNICATION IS CRITICAL to good patient care and to patient flow. Most times, an initial telephone call, often for an urgent need, sets the tone for a new patient's first impression of the practice. A smooth operational flow on each visit helps create a good experience for patients and increases the chances that they will return.

Triage Systems

In a medical practice, triage – prioritizing medical treatment based on urgency – is typically done by a triage nurse who handles patient calls related to questions or concerns. Many of the questions a patient typically asks can be answered by the nurse following specific protocols. Other questions may result in a patient requesting an appointment or asking for a nurse or physician follow-up call.

Triage systems can increase patient satisfaction and help the physicians to better manage their time. Typical triage systems include:

- Physician-approved guidelines for treatment;
- Procedures for documentation;

- Appropriate responses to calls about emergent, urgent, and nonurgent problems; and
- Guidelines for categorizing calls as life-threatening, urgent, important, and routine, and appropriate response times.

In most practices, nurses provide triage in an informal or a formal manner. Patients appreciate the ready availability of a nurse who can answer questions and take any appropriate action.

Written guidelines serve as training and procedural documents along with physician authorizations for releasing certain information. Triage calls are handled according to callers' symptoms and/or needs; appropriate protocols are specialty and symptom specific.

Every clinical phone call to the practice should be documented in a standard manner. Nurses today usually use some type of electronic telephone call form. They obtain the information and send it to the physician for physician comments. With an electronic medical record (EMR) system, a nurse or other employee accomplishes this function with the telephone messaging system. In any case, all telephone calls and advice given must be placed in patients' medical records.

Appropriate education and training of staff performing the triage function is essential. Triage staff must be qualified and able to assess a problem, provide information, and know when to refer the problem to the physician. The practice administrator must be comfortable with their judgment because ultimately the practice is liable for the advice given. Nurses perform most triage functions because they have the necessary skill level to evaluate medical problems.

◼ Call Coverage

Often, physicians may be responsible for their own call coverage from 7 a.m. on Monday morning until 5 p.m. on Friday afternoon. Typical call coverage includes:

- After-hours emergencies;
- Requests for prescription renewals;

- Patient questions; and
- Hospital rounds.

Call coverage for a group practice often depends on how many hospitals the physician covers. Small group practices usually designate one physician to take weekend call, with a second doctor identified as backup. Generally the backup physician was not assigned call the previous weekend – assuming the number of doctors in the group accommodates this rotation. In a larger practice, more physicians must be available to cover the larger patient base. Employment in a group does not necessarily mean the physicians take less call.

In regard to hospital call, the medical staff bylaws at each hospital the practice is affiliated with must be checked to determine how often the physicians are expected to be on call for unassigned emergency room duty.

Also, handling of communications among the physicians, the group's answering service, and the patient need to be clarified. Do physicians prefer to be paged by a beeper? Cellular phones now have a paging capacity, making communications more efficient.

An answering service experienced in helping medical practices is usually used to receive off-hours calls and route them to the appropriate after-hours triage nurse and/or on-call physician. This facilitates call coverage. The protocol typically includes having the primary incoming telephone line placed on call forwarding to the answering service each weekday evening and on Fridays for the weekend (unless weekend hours are offered). This will ensure that all patients, the emergency room, and the hospital have immediate access to the physician on call.

Medical Records

Every interaction with a patient must be documented. So a key component of a medical group practice is the medical records function. Throughout a physician's medical training, he or she has relied on the medical record and knows it as THE key to patient care. It presents the who, what, why, where, when, and how of patient care. It is the major communication tool for physicians in interfacing with patients, staff, and other physicians.

The medical record is a legal document; it captures information about clinical services. It is also an accounting document; it serves as the basis for billing. From the payer's perspective, if patient care was not documented, it was **not done**. Accuracy is the bottom line. Medical records are reviewed by outside organizations – insurance companies, malpractice carriers, and accreditation agencies. For all these reasons, it is critical that medical records be factual, clear, concise, legible, and timely.

Physician Responsibilities

The medical record can be an asset or a liability to the physician. If the physician ensures that each patient encounter is recorded quickly, accurately, and completely, this documentation will fulfill legal and payer requirements. If the physician does not complete the record by the end of the day, the accuracy of the record could be compromised. Completeness is also imperative. Omissions in the medical record fall upon the physician for proof. The payer requires documentation – correct documentation – before reimbursement. No documentation, no payment.

The office staff helps physicians learn about medical record documentation. For example, if a correction needs to be made in the record, a line should be drawn through the information in a way that one can still read through the line. Then make the correction, sign and date it.

Documentation Basics

As in hospitals, every patient has a separate medical record with the same standard data elements for each encounter. Each patient encounter must be signed by the provider.

Medical record progress notes include current vital signs and are presented in the SOAP format:

1. Subjective – complaints of patient;
2. Objective – observations and examination by provider;

3. <u>A</u>ssessment – diagnosis; and

4. <u>P</u>lan – actions to be taken.

The need to document seems obvious, but it is not unusual to find a progress note without a patient name. Each progress note should have a patient name and birth date.

Payment and charge information is stored in the billing/practice management system, not in the medical chart.

Paper Medical Records vs. Electronic Medical Records

Medical records can be maintained manually or through an electronic system. Paper medical records requirements include:

- Supplies – charts, dividers, progress notes, forms;
- Transcription;
- Filing system – alphabetic or numeric; and
- Storage.

A well-organized medical records department is critical to maintaining efficiency in patient care and reducing malpractice risks. A larger department is necessary to maintain a paper medical record system than an EMR. A poorly run department impacts every member of the staff, whereas a well-run department is hardly noticed.

Space for medical records and storage for purged paper records must be planned, but this can be costly for the practice. Groups often use outside storage facilities to conserve office space.

EMRs are definitely an option for group practices; they are feasible even for small practices. EMRs have a higher initial cost than paper records, but a lower operating cost because of lower staff and supply costs. Space needs often are less also.

Many physicians report that their encounter documentation is more complete with an EMR. Also, records are more readily available because there are no misfiled or lost records.

HIPAA Implications

The Health Insurance Portability and Accountability Act of 1996 has extensive compliance requirements related to medical records. For example, information may be released without consent for treatment, payment, and operational purposes. However, written consent from the patient is required to release information for any other reason.

Physicians must stay current and comply with HIPAA requirements. In addition, the medical records staff should be trained about the legal requirements for the release of medical information. A confidentiality statement and privacy policy should be included in the employee handbook. A breach of confidentiality can be grounds for immediate dismissal.

■ Supply Management

A topic often coupled with facility management is supply management. Both have clinical aspects essential for the running of a medical practice. Physicians will likely want to have a basic understanding of supply costs, inventory, and vendors as they join the practice.

Just consider the impact of supplies on the budget. The supply specialist in the practice typically will shop for the best prices. These may be available from a cooperative buying group or from the hospital where the physicians have privileges. Some supplies, like immunization vaccines, have expiration dates and high costs and therefore need special management.

Inventory control is vital. The administrator will want to know that there are enough supplies in stock – but not an excessive amount. It is expensive to store unneeded supplies and drugs that may expire. That's why supply specialists use just-in-time buying. They also tend to foster good relationships with several vendors so they get the best prices and best service.

For further information on controlling supplies, and in particular, pharmaceutical supplies, refer to Chapter 7.

Chapter 2 **Providing Relevant and Accurate Information to Patients**

■ Communication Systems

The needs, limitations, and requirements of those who use a particular communication system (e.g., voice mail, e-mail, electronic medical records) should be the #1 consideration. These requirements include defining the goals, expectations, and capabilities of the users of the communication system, including physicians, staff, patients, vendors, and any other stakeholder group that may require access to the practice. The sophistication of the communication system is often dependent on the level of sophistication of the users. If some users, such as elderly patients, are not computer literate, it is important to provide multiple avenues for communication to ensure that these patients can access the services provided by the practice.

The primary goal of patients is to have access to a communication system that allows them to communicate with the physician and the support staff as appropriate. Patients need to be able to make and change appointments, ask questions, obtain prescription renewals and referrals, request records, and discuss myriad other issues that are extremely important to the patient. Physicians and practice staff want a system by which they can communicate among themselves and with other health care providers and organizations, respond to patient requests, and attend to the normal business activities of the practice – and to do it all in an efficient and cost-effective manner.

Telephones and Voice Mail

The most obvious methods of communication include telephone, voice mail, fax, Internet, e-mail, pagers, and point-to-point delivery as serviced by the U.S. Postal Service, FedEx, UPS, and others. Each form of communication has its own purpose, which is normally derived from its individual strengths and weaknesses.

The most obvious and prevalent communication tool in use in practices is the telephone with voice mail capability. The strengths of the telephone lie primarily in its accessibility and its familiarity among all possible users. The telephone affords the user the opportunity to easily obtain live access to the target party. In the event that the desired recipient of the telephone communication is unavailable, the voice mail capability functions as an adequate, low-cost method of allowing the caller to leave messages for the recipient. The telephone system is limited only by the number of trunk lines that are installed and the number of personnel available to answer the calls.

In addition, the telephone can act as a marketing tool, providing information concerning the practice through a message-on-hold program that provides information concerning the practice. This message does need to be updated on a regular basis, such as every three to six months, to keep it from becoming stale and annoying to those individuals who call the practice on a regular basis. After normal office hours, the telephone can be forwarded to any number of answering services who can function as the physician's office in taking and forwarding the appropriate messages and calls to the on-call physician, thereby ensuring a patient's 24-hour access to medical support.

The weaknesses of this form of communication may, in some cases, seem contradictory to its strengths. Proper, detailed planning is again the best route to take to avoid or mitigate many of the weaknesses of a telephone system. This planning may include the use of call centers to receive and direct calls; defining call flow, including the use of hunt groups (a series of telephone lines identified as a group such that if one line is busy, the next available line is used – it "hunts" for the next line) and triage systems for handling inbound calls; developing answering standards; and handling emergency call protocols. Frustration among all of the users of the system will occur when a telephone system is not designed properly, resulting in calls that are not routed to the appropriate staff member, or when there are insufficient trunks to respond to the demand for access. Even where sufficient trunks exist, the lack of adequate numbers of properly trained staff to answer and respond to the volume of calls will also cause significant issues. Many users of telephone systems are intolerant of voice mail systems and are frustrated when calls are not returned on a timely basis. To reduce complaints concerning the use of voice mail systems, a practice needs to develop and implement detailed guidelines concerning expectations with regard to clearing and responding to voice mail messages. The use of auto-attendant and voice mail systems can become extremely confusing, especially for the elderly patient.

Websites

A relatively new communication tool being used by more and more practices and patients every day is through the development and implementation of Internet-based Websites and e-mail access. Through these sites, a practice can make its information available to a public made up of potential patients, referring physicians, and the community at large. Properly designed and publicized Websites also have the capability of reducing the volume of telephone calls received by an office by enabling existing patients to refill pharmaceuticals, request chart copies, download forms, obtain directions, and ask questions via e-mail. In addition to providing practice-specific information, Websites can provide medical education as well as links to other Websites concerning medical conditions and procedures that would otherwise result in telephone calls or extended office visits. Through the use of interactive programs located on a practice's Website, patients can become educated on

Example of Using a Website to Educate Patients

© 2008 Englewood Orthopedic Associates. Reprinted with permission.

surgical procedures being considered and the different types of clinical tests that the patient may receive. As this form of education can be accomplished at the patient's convenience, with respect to both time and location, it is a positive adjunct to the use of pamphlets, videotapes, and CDs. To be most effective, the Website should contain current, accurate information and be easy for the user to navigate (see Exhibit 1 for an example).

Internet

The use of the Internet also allows a practice to respond to and handle other clinical and administrative functions, including obtaining clinical information from such other providers as hospitals and imaging centers as well as making use of available telemedicine services, if appropriate, based on geographic location. The various administrative functions that can be accomplished through the use of the Internet include electronic submission of insurance claims, confirmation of a patient's insurance coverage, follow-up on previously submitted insurance claims, and Web-based conferencing. To accomplish these tasks, sufficient bandwidth and data ports should be available to the staff and physicians who would utilize these services.

To effectively use the technical methods of communication, it is the responsibility of the practice to ensure that all staff receives proper training in the utilization of these tools. Staff and physicians should receive sufficient training to become proficient and comfortable in the use of all of the software and technological tools that assist them in the performance of their duties. As new technologies (e.g., EHRs, intra-office e-mail, and automated patient notification systems) are introduced into the practice, the need to train affected personnel in areas of data and word processing increases. Some of the training in specific technology applications may require formal training sessions, whereas other modalities, such as reading manuals and online training, may also be utilized. Even after initial training takes place, policies should be established to ensure that periodic refresher training is provided so individual staff members remain proficient and up-to-date on the specifics of the technology tools they are using. In addition, as previously discussed, the Internet is an extremely powerful avenue to provide educational opportunities to patients through the use of interactive educational programs that can either reside on a practice's Website or be accessed through links to other medical educational sites on the Web.

Most physicians carry personal cell phones, but many still use pagers or cell phone/pagers to enable the office or answering service to reach them when they are not in the office. Although pagers can be effective in notifying a physician that he or she is needed, they are limited in that they do not allow for two-way communication. The physician or other recipient of the page may be required to call or otherwise respond to the page to confirm that the page has been received.

Fax and Deliveries

The two remaining methods of communication are the use of fax transmissions and door-to-door delivery, such as normal postal mail, otherwise known as "snail mail." While neither method is used to any great extent to communicate with patients, both methods are used for physicians and other health care providers (e.g., hospitals, clinical laboratories, and imaging centers) to transfer needed patient information in a secure manner. As with all other methods of communication, policies need to be developed that determine how mail and other packages are to be handled when reaching the practice but not the specific intended recipient. An example of this would be whether physicians open their own mail, or a member of the staff opens the mail and forwards to the physician only the items that require the physician's attention.

The constant growth and evolution within the field of communication have resulted in easier methods of contact among patients, physicians, and other health care providers. Medical practices and their leadership should continue to embrace this growth in technology to ensure continued, effective communication between patients and the medical practices.

Community Outreach Programs

Developing community outreach, public relations, and customer relations programs is unique because these tasks are intangible. When designing such programs, the medical practice must take into account the aesthetics and psychological benefits to the target audience. To develop appropriate plans and programs, the practice must first define the community in which it operates. By definition, a community is a group of people who share a particular situation, whether that situation is living in the same area, going to the same house of worship, or another defining group. Being part of a community induces a duty to one another. Medical practices have a duty to provide residents in their geographic area with the best-quality health care.

Patient Education

Patient education is an important part of a medical practice's community outreach that also helps in maintaining practice visibility. Brochures, newsletters, videos, and medical practice Websites are common methods for patient education. The quality and content of these materials must be considered to ensure that the practice's aims and positioning goals are accomplished. In addition, because of the advances of technology and communication, there is a wider range of media from which to communicate with patients.

Patient Handbooks

A simple method for patient communication is the use of patient handbooks. These handbooks can be easily printed in-house because of the advances in personal computers and software, or they can be purchased through vendors. The purpose of a patient handbook is to communicate important information to help patients and their families better understand the treatment and care process. Patient handbooks enable patients and their families to play essential roles in the treatment of disease.

Patient-Communication Protocols

Communication is of the utmost importance in treating patients and their illnesses. Often, during the course of medical treatment, patients and their families are thrust into new and confusing experiences. It is the duty of physicians to ensure that all patient communications are clear and effective.

Verbal communication is the primary method used to convey health information to patients about their diagnosis and treatment options; however, verbal communication is fraught with difficulty. Supplementing verbal communication with written information and instruction is an essential part of establishing effective patient-communication protocols. Written material affords a patient the opportunity to read and reflect upon information when opportune, not just when he or she consults with the physician. Written brochures are usually readily available from professional associations as well as online.[14]

Medical practice executives should clearly outline patient-communication protocols so that all patients will receive the information necessary to make informed treatment decisions. Protocols should establish step-by-step instructions and include methods to assess patient understanding of physician instructions. Use of effective communication protocols will ensure that patients are informed; thus, such procedures can also be an effective risk management strategy.

Leveraging Technology

The Internet and other advances in technology have enabled even the smallest medical practices to engage in the practice of telehealth. Telehealth, like telemedicine, uses technology to provide clinical and medical services over geographic distances, rather than by traditional face-to-face methods, in a timely and convenient manner. In addition, telehealth also uses technology to deliver nonclinical medical services, such as patient education and administrative functions.[15]

Telehealth typically employs the use of interactive video to treat and interact with patients. Other telehealth methods include online discussion forums for the purpose of consultations and the ongoing management of patients. Telehealth can also provide patients and clinical professionals with education and training opportunities.[16]

Brochures

Brochures can be an effective method of educating patients about illnesses and courses of treatment; however, they can be expensive to purchase and time-consuming to develop. On the positive side, brochures provide a written summary of what the patient needs to know about a particular procedure or condition. Studies have shown that informed patients are more likely to have better outcomes and require less staff time and attention.

An alternative to the printed brochure is to provide information via a medical practice Web page. Downloadable files can be used to transmit important information. An added advantage is the savings in printing costs, as well as the ability to update materials with little or no expense.

Community Focus and Collaboration

To be successful in today's health care environment, medical practices should have a defined strategy for interacting with the community. An organization's reputation, profitability, and even its continued existence can depend on the degree to which the community supports its efforts. By virtue of being health care providers, medical practices have an obligation to serve their communities. Therefore, it is critical for the medical practice executive to formulate a strategy to develop and maintain a community focus.

Awareness Building

One duty of medical practices is to build awareness of health issues impacting citizens. By virtue of collaborating with the community – both the citizenry and perhaps other medical practices – medical practices are able to actively involve those directly affected by certain issues. Collaboration in health initiatives enables co-learning, by which the community and medical practice contribute equally, and are thus able to achieve more than they would be able to do individually. Together, the partnership creates something new and valuable, thus creating a deeper commitment on behalf of all parties. Community collaborations help to "develop and maintain mutually respectful and dynamic partnerships with communities."[17]

Targeted Messages

Through the partnership synergy that results from deeply valuing one another's beliefs and knowledge, and through working in partnership with community residents, collaboration can help uncover the true needs of a community. Once these needs are identified, targeted messages can be developed to address any health problems that may exist. In addition, targeted health services can be developed to meet these needs as well.[18]

Cultural Sensitivity

Community collaboration can improve cultural sensitivity by virtue of working with disparate and diverse groups of people. When individuals come together to work on community problems, such as health problems, they learn to value the contributions of others, and hence to trust one another. In addition, individuals learn to value the differing perspectives that they previously did not. The value of the experiences obtained in collaborative work cannot be underestimated.

These experiences can help contribute to the cultural competency of the organization. By learning, understanding, and valuing cultural differences, practice patterns can be adjusted or reframed, so that treatment and health information can be delivered in a culturally acceptable manner.

Community Involvement

Community involvement is closely aligned with the mission of health care – to serve and help others. Thus, it is logical that individuals involved in health care would actively seek to participate in community activities and functions. Aside from this shared philosophy, it makes business sense to be a responsible member of the community.

Community involvement can be achieved through numerous methods. For instance, medical practices can sponsor health fairs to educate the local community regarding important health issues. Charitable care is also another way to interact with the local community. These experiences can also be leveraged through local media outlets; however, care should be taken so that media attention does not overshadow the charitable efforts.

■ Analysis of Community Health Risks

For a medical practice to meet the needs of the health care community, it has to ascertain what those needs are. To do so, a systematic process for describing and quantifying the risks associated with a particular health problem and the possible consequences should be established.[19] A step-by-step procedure can be utilized to conduct an assessment of the health risks present in a particular community. The first step is to define the health care community and identify key individuals and organizations. Particular attention should be given to achieving broad representation and include individuals with diverse viewpoints regarding problems and solutions.[20]

Engaging Partners

Medical practice executives need to develop creative and flexible methods to engage partners and community members in a conversation regarding community health risks. One strategy that may be employed is to schedule meetings at different times and locations, employing a variety of methods including town forums, conference calls, and anonymous surveys.[21]

Collecting Data

An excellent first step in the data collection process is to access community health data via community and state government Websites. Often, these Websites offer a plethora of secondary data, eliminating the need to collect firsthand or primary data. However, sometimes additional quantitative and qualitative data are necessary to present a complete picture of a particular community's health risks.[22]

Developing Health Priorities

Once data have been compiled and analyzed, the medical practice executive should engage community partners and members of the community in a stakeholder conversation to establish criteria so that priority areas can be identified. Once criteria have been established, the list of health risks present in the community can be ranked.[23]

Clarifying the Issue

To gain a clear understanding of the health risks, it is necessary to explore factors that contribute to the problem and determine which aspect of the problem is actually the area of concern. It is often necessary to collect additional data to understand the relationship between a health indicator, the available resources, and other influential factors.

Implementation Plan

Once this groundwork has been set, the medical practice executive should consider strategy and develop an implementation plan. Rather than reinventing the wheel, successful strategies utilized in other communities should be considered. The key to implementation is selecting a course of action that is manageable and evaluating the course of action to ensure success.

Wellness/Health Benchmarks

To judge the success of community health interventions, the medical practice executive should compare local results with national or state campaigns. One such national resource is Healthy People 2010, which is a comprehensive set of disease prevention and health promotion objectives for the nation to achieve by 2010.[24] In addition, most states have established health benchmarks for communities to achieve.

To assess the effectiveness of addressing community health risks, the medical practice executive can conduct periodic surveys and compare them to state- and national-level efforts. By comparing the results of local health care efforts with state and national surveys, behavioral change can be assessed. When gaps in progress are identified, efforts can be redirected to help achieve better disease management results.

Public Relations Methods

Just like other forms of marketing, public relations should also have a carefully structured plan. Effective methods for promoting a medical practice's name and services include conducting an open house, participating in speakers bureaus, authoring newspaper articles and columns, posting Website presentations, and creating physician referral newsletters.

Open Houses

Open houses provide an excellent reason to invite customers and referral sources to your medical group practice. Open houses can be used to introduce new physicians, highlight new services, or celebrate a milestone within the medical practice. Members of the media from the local newspaper as well as radio and television stations should be included so that good relationships can be established. Establishing positive relationships with media outlets is essential in being able to leverage and influence present and future media coverage.[25]

Speakers Bureaus

Participating in speakers bureaus can be an effective part of a medical practice's public relations efforts. Speakers bureaus present the opportunity to communicate the practice's marketing message to a captive audience. Often, speaking engagements are publicized and covered by the media, increasing their value as a public relations tool.[26]

Newspaper Columns

The printed word is an effective method to support public relations activities. Newspapers provide a cost-free forum for medical practice executives and physicians to share their opinions and expertise to the community at large.

Website Presentations

Using the Internet for advertising and promoting a medical practice has become commonplace. Developing a Website helps the practices to describe its offerings and also delivers the message that the organization is up-to-date and on the cutting edge. Done properly, Website presentation can be an effective tool for exposure.

Physician Referral Newsletters

Fact sheets, physician referral newsletters, and brochures can be tailored to support public relations. Printed material provides the necessary facts about the medical practice and its services to prospective clients as well as to other physicians who may be unaware of the practice's offerings. Brochures can be created and printed in-house so that costs can be reduced and the content can be easily changed as necessary.

Publicity

Publicity refers to free communication of information about an organization's facility and available services, which is an integral part of the organization's public relations strategy. Because publicity is free, this method for reaching the community and customers should be leveraged.

Opportunities for publicity can be categorized into three general areas:

1. News releases;
2. Media coverage; and
3. Medical media opportunities.

News Releases

The media plays an important informational role in community outreach opportunities. Members of the local media are continually searching for public health information activities as part of their public service mission.[27]

Medical group practices can develop news releases by partnering with the local media to highlight events occurring at the facility, or perhaps to highlight outstanding staff members. For example, a practice may want to develop a news release showcasing new technology that the practice offers, or perhaps a physician who received a national recognition award.

Media Coverage

An excellent method to ensure media coverage is to identify human interest stories. Medical practice executives need to be creative and identify events that are of interest to the community. One such event may be how staff members are participating in charity work, such as physicians volunteering at local charities providing health care to the homeless and uninsured. Another example may include media coverage of a health fair sponsored by the medical practice. Further means to generate media coverage can be accomplished by organizing programs and special events to which the public is invited.[28]

Medical Media Opportunities

It is important for the medical practice executive to leverage media opportunities to help market the practice's services. Some opportunities include working with local radio and television stations to provide medical information, or celebrating and taking advantage of nationally recognized efforts, such as Patient Safety Awareness Week or American Heart Month, by creating and/or sponsoring public service announcements with local media outlets. Another cost-free method is encouraging clinical staff members to write editorials and op-ed pieces for local papers and newsletters.[29]

Chapter 3 **Developing and Implementing a Referral Management Process**[30]

◢ The Value of Relationships Beyond Your Patients

The quality and depth of your relationships have the power to drive every aspect of your business:

- Great relationships with your physicians can result in easier compliance with challenges such as dictation and documentation. It will also result in a greater willingness to consider your ideas as you work together to grow and refine the practice.

- Strong relationships with your employees will increase their willingness to go over and above the call of duty. It will reduce tardiness, absences, and the waste of practice resources. It will reduce turnover and increase productivity.

- Great relationships with vendors can bring extraordinary resources and opportunities to your practice – from additional free samples to free food and incentives for staff to inclusion in beta-site studies and new product trials.

- Strong relationships with referral sources can mean the difference between a struggling practice and a burgeoning one.

There is no marketing tool or promotion that is more powerful than a great relationship. Take the time to evaluate and take greater stock in your key relationships. The return on your investment of time and attention will be healthy growth, meaningful interactions, and the long-term success of your practice.

Fostering Positive Referral Relationships

Now that you understand the value of relationships in general, let's talk about some specific behaviors that can foster positive referral relationships.

A good way to begin is to make sure your physicians are accessible and friendly to primary care physicians – in the medical staff lounge, at grand rounds, at committee meetings, and at social outings. Encourage them also to look for opportunities to provide in-service presentations regarding a new technique or service to the staff of primary care physicians in your area.

In many communities, physical growth impacts physicians' abilities to know colleagues as they did 20 years ago. Communities are more spread out geographically, as well as sometimes in medical practice towers. Nevertheless, it remains important to track referring physicians. And after you know who they are, you have a chance to acknowledge their referral patterns to you.

Studies show that referring physicians expect communication about the patients they refer to you, of course, but they also want to know you appreciate the referral. Communicating also helps to maintain your group's professional relationships. This is enhanced when you develop and implement a plan to keep in touch with them (see Exhibit 2).

Here are some suggestions that will help you accomplish this.

- Spend time with referrers. Find out what's going on in their practices;
- Send brief, periodic updates when your group adds locations, services, products, or new physicians;
- Hold an open house for referral physicians' staff;

- Partner with a hospital or local university to conduct a continuing medical education program;

- Send letters introducing new practice associates and areas of the subspecialization they bring to your practice;

- Partner with a referring physician group to present informational talks at community groups;

- Volunteer for medical staff committees;

- Serve on community advisory boards and task boards relating to health in your community;

- Develop patient education materials about subjects that reflect the skill, knowledge, and interest of your group and distribute them to health professionals;

- Be visible and available;

- Encourage every physician in your group to do one promotional activity per month (minimum), such as taking a referring physician to lunch or dinner;

- Make referrers feel as if they're part of the team – report to them promptly and send their patients back to them;

- Send a thorough response – a detailed, diagnostic report – for every referral. Include an executive summary at the beginning of the report;

- Be available to referring doctors. Set aside a specific time every day to return calls;

- Schedule referred patients as quickly as possible. Set aside a block of time each day for this purpose – and let referrers know about it;

- Hold an annual educational seminar about your specialty. Arrange for continuing medical education credits;

- Make sure regular referrers know that they are important to you. Stay in touch and thank them regularly with a note or small gift or invite them to a special event; and

- Thank the staff of referrers by doing something special for one office each month. Send an appropriate gift to the office or have your staff take their staff to lunch.

In addition to these suggestions, there are other things you can do that will be of value to referring physicians. You should make it

---

EXHIBIT 2.
Referral Enhancement Behaviors for Physicians

Be Respectful of the Referrer

If you find something questionable about the patient's treatment, take it up privately with the referring physician. Unless it's medically necessary, don't repeat tests already performed, because this drives up costs and can be offensive to the referring physician as well as the patient.

Use Basic Marketing Techniques

Print your cell phone and e-mail address on your business cards that will be used specifically for your referring physicians to make it easy to reach you and your practice. Provide referrers with brochures that will be of value to their patients. Be sure to include a brochure rack to keep the referrer's office neat.

Monitor Your Referral Patterns

Keep a log of who is referring and check it every month. If you discover that referrals from certain colleagues are declining, call to find out if you or your practice has offended them in some way.

Remember Those Who Support Your Practice

It's not out of line to send a note or a gift certificate or to hose referrers who have helped build your practice. You may send lunch to a referral physician's office, host a referrer's staff to a wine and cheese evening in your office, or make a contribution in honor of physicians in your community.

Recognize That Referred Patients Are Ambassadors of Your Practice

When patients return to the primary physician and are appreciative of the referral, it helps to build positive relations on your behalf. Create systems within your practice to see referred patients on time, treat them respectfully, and communicate appropriately with referring physicians.

easy for them and their patients to use your services. If you joined a managed care panel after their booklet was printed, write a personal letter and let referrers know you're accessible and interested in their referrals. It's a perfect opportunity to let them know you set aside a few time slots every day for referred patients. Also let your top referrers know that you understand that when they need help, they need it now, not in two weeks.

At the same time, be sure to respect a referring physician's schedule. Rather than calling about a patient, you may want to consider other options. For example, information can be faxed or e-mailed, and both can be printed and added to the patient's chart as well.

Whether or not your physicians call a referring physician to report findings and recommendations, make sure they always send a prompt follow-up letter. And one important issue that's been learned from conducting numerous referral surveys: referrers appreciate having an executive summary of findings with the report.

If your practice follows a patient for a long time, keep the referring physician informed about the patient's progress. If you find it necessary to refer the patient to another physician, let the primary practice know. Most referring physicians will be annoyed if they're not informed that one of their patients has had surgery or hospitalization. It can be very embarrassing if the patient's family calls the primary doctor and he or she has no idea what is taking place.

Referring physicians usually have spent years developing relationships with their patients. They know they'll be called to help the family sort through issues and complications. For that reason, always engage and partner with the referring physician to plan case management.

In addition to showing respect for the referring physician, find a way to say thank you for the continual interaction between your two practices. You can do this by writing a personal note of thanks, making a phone call to express your appreciation, or simply initiating a gesture that communicates your awareness of the relationship your practices share.

Whenever possible and appropriate, remind your physicians to be sensitive when talking to referred patients – frequently, what your physicians say will be repeated to the primary doctors. An offhand remark or thoughtless statement may come back to haunt your practice.

Some specialists take the attitude that they're fixing a problem the primary care doctor can't solve. That certainly is not conducive to building positive referral relationships. Obviously, it's better for practice-building if the specialist realizes this and, instead, positions for a complementary relationship.

Remember, everybody benefits when referring relationships are open, honest, and interactive.

Chapter 4 **Designing Efficient Patient Flow Patterns to Maximize Physician Schedules**

FOR A PRACTICE TO BE EFFICIENT and allow the physician and staff to focus on patient care, attention should be paid to how work flows within the organization. This workflow, from a patient's perspective, includes the four primary steps of (1) making an appointment, (2) entering the office, (3) receiving treatment from the physician, and, finally, (4) leaving the office as a satisfied recipient of high-quality medical care.

In addition to patient-centered workflow are other distinctly separate workflows for business and clinical processes that do not directly affect, nor are they seen by, the patient. Analysis of patient flow should be undertaken, including the posting of charges and payments, filing of medical records, and processing of medical record copy requests. Examples of this type of analysis as applied to the first stage of the patient-centered and business workflows are shown in Exhibits 3 and 4.[31] Although patients do not see the behind-the-scenes workflows, they are affected by any breakdowns that occur within these flows. A significant portion of patient satisfaction with the practice is

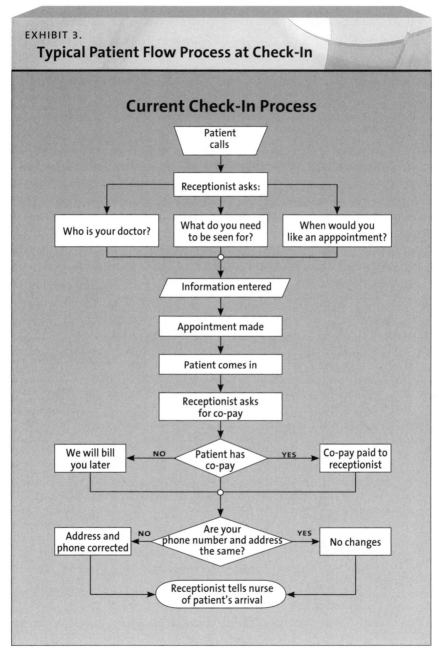

EXHIBIT 3.
Typical Patient Flow Process at Check-In

Current Check-In Process

Patient calls

↓

Receptionist asks:

Who is your doctor? | What do you need to be seen for? | When would you like an apppointment?

↓

Information entered

↓

Appointment made

↓

Patient comes in

↓

Receptionist asks for co-pay

↓

We will bill you later ← NO — Patient has co-pay — YES → Co-pay paid to receptionist

↓

Address and phone corrected ← NO — Are your phone number and address the same? — YES → No changes

↓

Receptionist tells nurse of patient's arrival

© 2004 Medical Group Management Association. Adapted with permission.

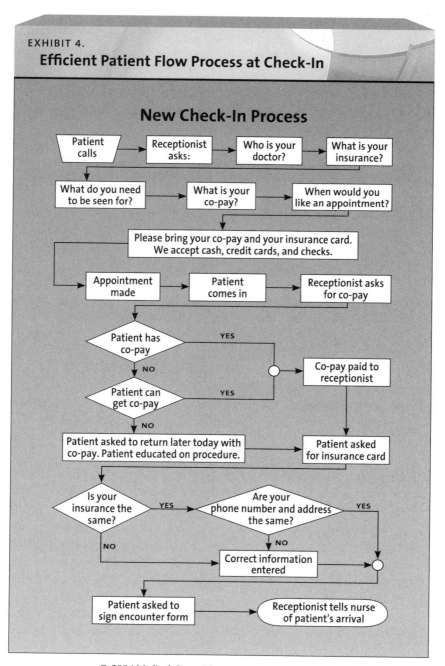

EXHIBIT 4.
Efficient Patient Flow Process at Check-In

New Check-In Process

Patient calls → Receptionist asks: → Who is your doctor? → What is your insurance? → What do you need to be seen for? → What is your co-pay? → When would you like an appointment? → Please bring your co-pay and your insurance card. We accept cash, credit cards, and checks. → Appointment made → Patient comes in → Receptionist asks for co-pay → Patient has co-pay

Patient has co-pay — YES → Co-pay paid to receptionist
Patient has co-pay — NO → Patient can get co-pay — YES → Co-pay paid to receptionist
Patient can get co-pay — NO → Patient asked to return later today with co-pay. Patient educated on procedure.

Co-pay paid to receptionist → Patient asked for insurance card

Patient asked to return later today with co-pay. Patient educated on procedure. → Is your insurance the same? — YES → Are your phone number and address the same? — YES
Is your insurance the same? — NO → Correct information entered
Are your phone number and address the same? — NO → Correct information entered

Patient asked to sign encounter form → Receptionist tells nurse of patient's arrival

© 2004 Medical Group Management Association. Adapted with permission.

determined by the efficiency, accuracy, and effectiveness of the steps that are accomplished behind the scenes.

The framework or initial anticipated flow for patient activity is determined by the day's schedule of appointments. "Good scheduling demands good planning, good data, good information systems, and, above all, good staff; that is, workers who are trained, committed, and empowered to provide top-notch customer service."[32] To properly develop an appointment schedule that allows the provider to be efficient, and to anticipate staffing needs, the development of patient demand projections based on several factors, including patient demand variations, should be conducted based on the day of the week and time of day; age of patients, which can affect the amount of time needed for the provider/patient interaction; and the specialty and personality of the physician, which can also affect the amount of time needed for the provider/patient interaction.

Other factors that can affect a daily schedule, but cannot be as easily projected, include emergencies; calls from hospitals, nursing homes, and other physicians; and last-minute cancellations and no-shows. Some of these issues can be anticipated, and schedule modifications and office procedures can be implemented in an effort to reduce their negative effects. A variety of different scheduling methodologies can be used to alleviate some of these variations. The scheduling methodology that would alleviate these concerns to the greatest degree would be a block schedule, as discussed previously, by which several patients are told to come in at the same time (e.g., on the hour) and are seen based on their time of arrival. This method does reduce the issues of gaps and providers waiting for delayed and no-show patients, but it also increases patient waiting time.[33] To reduce the risk of no-shows, staff can be assigned or computer systems implemented to call patients to remind them of their appointments, appointment slots can be held open to allow for last-minute add-ons, and the judicious use of double booking can be implemented to compensate for last-minute cancellations and no-shows that do occur.

Issues that may upset or aggravate patients during the patient workflow cycle may include extensive delays in the waiting room, not being advised to bring specific documents with them to the appointment with the physician, extended waiting times in the examination room, and the inability to get timely follow-up appointments when leaving the offices of the practice. Many of these outcomes can be avoided by simple patient communication. When confirming appointments, practices should remind patients of the documents and forms that they should bring to their appointments. Many of these forms are unique to specific insurance carriers (e.g., Medicare, Medicaid, employer plans, and commercial carriers), and plans and may include referrals and procedure precertifications. Communicating with the patient, explaining what is going on, and reassuring the patient can usually mitigate any annoyance or aggravation on the patient's part. Sufficient time should also be included within each visit to allow the physician to dictate notes and to respond to issues that become known during the visit with the patient.

The clinical flow within a practice is integral to ensuring that patients receive effective and efficient care. Clinical flow begins long before the patient arrives in the practice's offices. Examination rooms need to be stocked, preferably in a standardized manner, with the supplies that may be required by the physician or staff. By standardizing both the items to be stored in each examination room and their locations within each examination room, staff will be able to reduce the amount of time needed to search for a specific everyday item. An alternative to maintaining stocks of supplies within each examination room is the use of small supply rooms or cabinets close to several examination rooms. Although potentially increasing the walking required of the clinical support staff, this method of maintaining supply stocks will reduce the overall amount of supplies that need to be maintained in inventory.

Medical records need to be retrieved and reviewed before the patient's arrival to ensure that all test results are available and that any required instruments or testing materials are available for the physician's use. Preplanning each visit and ensuring that the required information and supplies are available can reduce the amount of time needed for each visit, thereby enabling the physician to be more efficient in the use of his or her time.

Upon arrival, the patient begins the direct, on-site involvement by checking in at the practice's reception desk. At that time, the patient is identified and greeted by the reception staff. A new patient is normally asked to complete various intake documents providing the demographic and billing/insurance information that the practice needs to initiate a medical record and bill the appropriate source for payment. An established patient will normally be asked to confirm the information on file to ensure that no changes have taken place since the last office visit. The patient may then be asked to provide copayment and any referral documents that may be appropriate. After completion of the required paperwork, a member of the clinical support staff normally escorts the patient to an examination room.

In addition to the direct hands-on care provided by both the physician and the clinical staff for the patient are several other areas within the clinical encounter that may require action by the physician or staff. These tasks, based on the needs of the patient, may include:

1. Developing and documenting a treatment plan that addresses the patient's medical needs;

2. Providing needed educational support to the patient, which may include reviewing a videotape or providing printed material on the issues that concern the patient;

3. Ensuring that the patient has provided informed consent for procedures that are being scheduled;

4. Addressing human immunodeficincy virus and other communicable-disease issues that may be of concern to the patient and others; and

5. Initiating any referrals or other carrier-required documents that may be needed by the patient to obtain the care indicated in the plan of treatment.

After providing the services that are required by the patient, the remainder of the clinical workflow for the staff consists of escorting the patient from the examination area and cleaning and preparing the examination room for the next patient. For the patient, the final step is check-out, where he or she will receive the required documents and forms, make any future appointments with the practice, and pay for any financial amounts that may be due and were not collected at time of check-in. For the physician, the final part of the clinical workflow process is made up of properly documenting the patient history, the clinical services provided, and the plan for future services. The last step for the physician – determining the procedure and diagnostic codes to be used to categorize this patient's visit – begins the second half of the business workflow process.

The business workflow identifies, collects, and processes all of the information required to properly and accurately bill for the services rendered by the practice. The business workflow begins when the patient calls to make the first appointment with the physician. At the time of making that first appointment, the practice should begin the process of obtaining the demographic information concerning the patient. This demographic information includes name, address, telephone number, guarantor, insurance information, and employer. At this time, the practice will normally confirm that the practice participates in the patient's insurance plan. The collection of demographic information continues when the patient arrives at the practice and provides a copy of an insurance card and, if appropriate, a referral from a primary care physician, and completes and signs the documents required by the practice. These documents normally include an intake registration form that details all of the patient's demographic information, a medical history, an authorization to assign the patient's insurance benefits to the practice, and a confirmation that the patient has been advised of the practice's Health Insurance Portability and Accountability Act (HIPAA) policies.

The procedure and diagnostic codes that the physician determines upon completion of the appointment will be used to categorize the services rendered. In many practices, this information is provided on a paper form that may variously be called a charge ticket, routing sheet, or trip ticket. This form will also indicate the additional billable services provided by either the physician or the support staff. These services may include immunizations or other injectable medications, X-rays, splints, or clinical laboratory services. In practices that use an electronic health record, the proper procedure codes may be generated directly from the physician's notes and posted to the patient's account within the practice management system.

It is this code determination that initiates the second phase of the business workflow. During this phase of the business workflow, the process of billing and collection takes place. The patient's insurance is reviewed and the required co-payment is collected, although in many offices this portion of the process is accomplished before the patient sees the physician. The determination of when the co-pay is collected is often a function of the physical layout of the office. The charge ticket is then reviewed for completeness, and the charges and the copayment received are posted to the patient's account. Some offices post the charges in batches, whereas other offices post them as each patient leaves the office. There is no specific right or wrong way, as it is totally dependent on the workflow design within the specific office and the volume of visits and services. At the end of each day, the posted batches of charges and payments received are closed out, meaning that all charge tickets and payments are accounted for and posted. The remaining business process consists of transmitting the charges to the appropriate third-party payers, applying the payments received from these payers to the appropriate patient account, posting any applicable contractual adjustments, and finally billing the patient or secondary insurance for any remaining balance. Interspersed within this process are the needs to respond to carrier requests for additional information, to appeal carrier denials of coverage or incorrect application of billing guidelines, and to respond to patient questions and requests for assistance in complying with the demands of the insurance carrier.

Throughout the process, and at all subsequent times, the practice must take all steps necessary to ensure patient confidentiality with respect to the medical treatment and status. All staff should be trained in the requirements of HIPAA regulations, and employee policies need to be specific in communicating the expectations of the practice that patient confidentiality is paramount within the organization.

Chapter 5

Maximizing the Patient Encounter[34]

Good communication is critical to good patient care and to patient flow. Telephone calls, scheduling, and patient registration set the tone for a patient's impression of the practice. A smooth operational flow on each visit helps create a good experience for patients and increases the chances that they will return.

◢ Patient Flow Patterns

A smooth operational flow on office visits from check-in to check-out creates a better experience for the patient and brings that patient back to the practice. From a business perspective, it is a bottom-line necessity for the practice. Efficient patient flow is the only way to maximize the practice's most important asset – the physician's time. It is the fundamental service/revenue equation: physician serves patient; patient care generates revenue.

Patient flow encompasses all the steps in the patient care sequence. It involves the best telephone usage, appropriate scheduling, efficient registration and check-in, satisfactory waiting experience, effective patient care in the exam room, and smooth check-out.

Physicians will focus on the clinical highlight of the patient flow sequence – the actual physician/patient encounter. However, it's important for the practice manager to understand all the parts of patient flow. Preparation and follow-up by staff ensure that the exam encounter goes smoothly.

The next sections will spotlight key operational elements including:

- Telephone usage and protocols;
- Scheduling;
- Registration/check-in and waiting; and
- Check-out.

Telephone Usage

Effective practice managers know that communications are critical to good patient care and that the telephone plays a key part in this vital function. Effective use of the telephone for scheduling, referrals, patient triage, answering patient questions, ordering and renewing prescriptions, handling insurance claims, and ordering supplies is mandatory for an efficient practice. Today, the phone often is just a part of a telecommunications system that includes use of the Internet and e-mail for many of these tasks. However, the phone continues to play a major part in practice communications.

Telephone systems range from the simple to the complex. The needs of the practice dictate the choice of system. A three-physician practice does not need the same system as a multiphysician, multisite practice. Systems now available offer a variety of features including automated attendant, call forwarding, call holding, speed dialing, conference calling, call park and pickup, voice paging, call transferring, voice mail, and others.

All of these options can increase practice efficiency. For example, automated attendants, which answer and route calls after prompting the patient, are now standard in many practices. An automated attendant does the work of a full-time-equivalent employee by routing calls to the appropriate source without human intervention. Typically no more than five options are offered; more can frustrate callers. Such options include:

- Schedule an appointment;
- Speak with a triage nurse (discussed in Chapter 1);
- Discuss a bill;

- Refill a prescription; and
- Speak with an operator.

Telephone Protocols

Telephone protocols are typically used to help staff make/answer low-urgency calls without consulting a physician. Such protocols include:

- Answering all calls within a standard number of rings (e.g., two) and repeating a standard greeting;
- Accepting and handling appointment calls courteously;
- Handling emergency calls calmly and quickly;
- Directing calls from hospitals and physicians appropriately;
- Responding to routine billing questions competently; and
- Referring employee personal calls graciously.

Patient Scheduling

Nearly every practice has the same pattern for patient flow – at least initially. The patient calls for an appointment, arrives for the appointment and checks in, is seen by a physician, and then the patient leaves. Scheduling begins the process.

Effective scheduling requires efficient planning, accurate and complete data, excellent information systems, and competent staff. Poor scheduling upsets patients, frustrates staff, reduces physician productivity, and erodes revenue. Proper scheduling ensures patient access to care, which is a concern to payers and measured by them via patient surveys. Improper scheduling can also generate malpractice concerns if patients feel they are not getting timely access to care. In summary, patient scheduling is a critical component of practice operations, patient satisfaction, and physician efficiency.

Schedule protocols impact numerous administrative and clinical performance matters; for example, who handles the scheduling. It can be done by the person answering the phone or by specific intake specialists, or the responsibility can be shared. In any case, thorough training and cross-training must be provided to anyone handling this task.

There are three general methods of scheduling:

1. **Single intervals:** Each visit receives the same amount (e.g., 15 minutes) on the scheduling calendar, regardless of the type of visit or patient complaint.

2. **Multiple intervals:** The intervals between appointments (e.g., 15–30 minutes) depend on the type of visit (e.g., new) or the patient complaint (e.g., health check).

3. **Block intervals:** A single block of time (e.g., on the hour and half hour) is established for multiple appointments regardless of the visit type or patient complaint. Scheduling several patients to arrive at the same time decreases any "down" time for the physician because there are always patients available to be seen. But it increases patient wait times as some patients must wait from the time they arrive until the other patients in that time block are seen.

Most practices use multiple intervals because it allows them to estimate the amount of time a patient may need and to balance this with patient waiting time.

Other approaches include:

- *Individual scheduling,* which provides a time slot for each patient. A no-show or late arrival affects the entire schedule. The physician loses time if the patient has to be rescheduled.

- *Modified wave scheduling,* which clusters patients at the beginning of each hour or block of time, followed by individual appointments every 10, 15, or 20 minutes during the rest of the hour or block. Specific types of appointments can be scheduled at certain time periods depending on the length of time of those appointments. For example, two sick-patient appointments would follow one for a physical exam. The medical assistant can room one patient while the physician sees another. This distributes patient flow evenly through the physician's day and decreases patient wait time.

- *Open access scheduling,* which is built on having open slots when the day begins so that a patient can be seen the same day as he or she calls. If the patient requests an appointment on another day, s/he is scheduled accordingly. Depending on the medical specialty, 30 percent to 50 percent of the appointments remain open for same-day calls. Open-access scheduling allows today's work to be done today. It also increases patient satisfaction because patients can be seen the same day they call for an appointment.

As every new practice manager soon learns, scheduling is a complex and ever-challenging task. Practices will experience patients who do not appear for the appointment (no-shows), patients who are habitually or occasionally late, and patients or staff with emergencies. Plans and protocols must anticipate such situations so there is the least impact possible to patient flow.

One scheduling challenge occasionally arises – how to deal appropriately with disabled individuals. Physicians cannot refuse to treat a patient because of his or her disabilities. For example, a practice cannot refuse to treat a patient with human immunodeficiency virus or acquired immunodeficiency syndrome, conditions protected under the Americans with Disabilities Act (ADA). Similarly, a physician's practice can't refuse to treat a person with a hearing impairment because it can't or doesn't want to pay for interpreter services. However, a practice can refuse to treat a patient because of specialty or current patient load.

The ADA mandates that a medical organization must provide, at its expense, auxiliary aids such as qualified interpreters, Braille materials, and large-print materials. More expensive auxiliary aids may not be required if they create an "undue burden." The ADA makes allowances for an undue burden that results in "significant difficulty or expense." What constitutes undue burden for a small practice vs. a large practice will differ. Undue burden is determined on a case-by-case basis.

Registration Process and Patient Check-In

When the patient arrives for an appointment, the registration process is an important part of how that person views a practice. Employees who greet patients and make eye contact, collect patient insurance and demographic information promptly, and enter it into the patient record system accurately help a practice run smoothly and collect all the income it is due.

The check-in experience begins the moment the patient opens the door. Put yourself in the position of the patient. What do you see? The reception area/waiting room space forms the patient's impression of the practice. The area should present an updated, well-lit décor, and have adequate and comfortable seating. An outdated, dirty, cluttered waiting room gives a negative impression of the entire practice. Even magazines several months old can convey an outdated image. Amenities such as fish tanks, and even a television with a VCR or DVD player, are often appropriate and make the waiting time seem to go faster.

The reception area is also one place to ensure there are no office design barriers for people with disabilities. Architectural barrier regulations address many physical aspects that allow accommodation of those with disabilities, such as handicap-accessible restrooms, access to the building (e.g., ramps to navigate stairs, elevators, automated doors) and parking set aside for the disabled. Any new construction must meet ADA standards. Practice managers should regularly review their office space to ensure that it offers easy access for people with disabilities.

Reception staff should be able to see and monitor the waiting areas so they can help any patient with special needs. A patient may become ill or highly anxious while waiting, so a clear view of these areas is critical. Patients will become upset if they have to wait longer than they think they should. So a practice often posts a sign stating its waiting time goal – usually no more than 20 minutes. This helps set patient expectations. If the schedule gets off-track (e.g., a physician was delayed at the hospital or a patient took extra time), the receptionist can communicate that fact to patients. Close to the reception area should be a private area to discuss personal financial matters such as payment issues.

Particular attention should be paid to how the reception area is designed to ensure patient confidentiality. The Health Insurance Portability and Accountability Act of 1996 (HIPAA) makes compliance of paramount importance and this must be considered in office design. The reception area is a place where inadvertent breaches of confidentiality can occur. Two staff members may discuss a patient and not notice that others in the area can overhear. Hallways, restrooms, and clinical areas are also areas where confidentiality is sometimes forgotten. Prudent practice managers help all staff to remember privacy concerns.

In a busy practice, the receptionist often forgets to look up when a patient enters and the patient feels invisible and unwelcome. Such a nongreeting may be a sign of an understaffed front desk and should be corrected. The role of receptionist is similar to that of a juggler. Not only do these staff members set the scene and the mood for the incoming patient, they also have many tasks to complete quickly and accurately. They must:

- Ensure the reception area stays attractive and comfortable;
- Greet each patient with enthusiasm and respect;
- Pay attention to patients during the registration process so they feel welcome and not like they're interrupting;
- Protect the patient's privacy with appropriate confidentiality procedures (e.g., sign-in methods);
- Be sensitive to the practice's waiting-time goal (e.g., 20 minutes) and inform patients of the reason for any delays; and
- Collect accurate, up-to-date clinical and billing information.

Information Collection

Efficient and accurate gathering of patient demographic and insurance information will help a practice run smoothly during the patient's visit and during the billing process. Inaccurate or incomplete information will lead to delayed processing of claims or even denials instead of reimbursement. To ensure that patient registration proceeds smoothly and accurately:

- Train receptionists to collect up-to-date information and confirm it for accuracy;
- Review forms for gathering patient information for completeness of questions asked and ease of use;
- Gather a patient's information prior to his or her appointment whenever possible to increase the efficiency of the

EXHIBIT 5.

Reviewing Accuracy of Patient Registration Process

	Yes	No
Do the staff accurately gather patient information including: ■ Name, address, phone number, and social security number; ■ Employment information; ■ Guarantor information; and ■ Insurance information, including copayment and expiration date?		
Are appropriate forms signed and dated, including: ■ Financial guarantee; ■ Authorization to treat; and ■ Other required forms?		

patient's actual visit and to review the insurer's copayments and coverage policies; and

■ Confirm the patient's address and insurance information with each visit.

Exhibit 5 is a checklist for reviewing the accuracy of the patient registration process.

The office manager will need to ensure that all necessary forms are stocked and the staff is trained to use them correctly.

Patient Check-Out

The patient's visit is not finished after the provider completes the exam or other service. It is up to the physician and/or practice employees to ensure that the patient understands any follow-up steps that must be taken, such as an X-ray or a laboratory test. If

EXHIBIT 6.

Completion of Patient Check-Out Process

	Yes	No
Does the patient understand preauthorization or referral request processes?		
Are copayments collected at registration or at the end of the appointment?		
Does the staff discuss the payment options that are available to the patient (credit cards, cash, checks)?		

additional services or a referral are recommended, the patient must understand what is required to obtain a preauthorization or a referral from the payer and who will complete those steps. The patient must understand what the insurer will cover and what he or she will be expected to pay for additional services. The practice must also obtain payment from the patient to cover the copayment or other charges incurred that day, if this was not done during check-in.

Exhibit 6 is a checklist for completing the patient's check-out process.

Chapter 6 **Maximizing Patient Satisfaction and Customer Care**[35]

Baseline Service Assessment

The first step toward knowing where to go is to be sure of where you are. A baseline service assessment examines how well the practice's external and internal customers are being served, including, but not limited to:

- **A patient survey** conducted at regular intervals and designed to provide relevant feedback from the patients' perspective;

- **Mystery patient assessments,** in which experienced professionals probe beyond the survey data to evaluate the specific performance dimensions that affect patient satisfaction;

- **Key-person interviews** to obtain input from the physicians and employees who work directly with patients and have the best ideas on how to improve service levels; and

- **Related performance indicators** that affect patient satisfaction, including staff turnover rates, requests for records transfer, trends in referrals from other physicians, anecdotal patient complaints, malpractice claims, and other data that measure the service strengths and weaknesses of the practice.

◼ Patient Satisfaction Survey

Because the business depends on patient loyalty and word-of-mouth referrals, patients are the practice's best source of information about what works well and what needs to be improved. A patient survey is the best tool for asking them what they think of the practice.

Patient surveys used to be optional; if a practice wanted to know what patients were thinking about the practice and its people, a survey was a good way to find out. Sometimes, owing to human nature, the surveys were "whitewash jobs" designed to produce high marks so as not to offend physicians and employees.

That was then. Today, in our competitive marketplace, knowing where the practice stands with patients and caregivers is imperative, and managers who "fudge" the findings are underserving the practice.

A poorly designed survey shortchanges patients, too, because unrealistic data may not produce the improvements that would benefit them. That's why much study has gone into how surveys are constructed, how best to distribute them, what kind of reports are most helpful to practice leaders and managers, and how survey data can help set priorities for improving the work processes and physician/staff service performance that affects patient satisfaction and referrals.

◼ Survey Design and Layout

Surveys are not perfect instruments. They are based on perceptions, which makes it difficult, even impossible, to set quantified norms for measuring performance.

The inability to set quantified criteria is a pitfall of many patient satisfaction surveys. For example, the survey instrument might ask, "In the last 12 months, how often did your visits to this doctor's office start within 15 minutes of your appointment?" Aiming for a quantifiable response does not take into account the inherent variability of patient expectations – one person can be dissatisfied with a 10-minute wait, while another may be content to sit for 30 minutes or longer in the reception area. If the purpose is to measure satisfaction, a practice is less interested in the length of the wait than in whether the patient was satisfied with the waiting time.

So what should the practice's patient survey look like? The questions are arranged to follow the patient's experience during the encounter as closely as possible, from making an appointment to checking out after the visit.

First, the questions must be stated as briefly and as clearly as possible. That's to ensure face validity (that is, the respondent understands what the question is about and gives an answer related to the performance dimension being rated) and content validity (that is, the questions are grouped together in a manner reflecting what actually happens during the encounter).

In a Medical Group Management Association (MGMA)-Sullivan/Luallin survey in *Star-Studded Service: Six Steps to Winning Patient Satisfaction*,[36] the questions are divided into five sections:

1. Access (making appointments, check-in, and waiting times);

2. Staff performance (reception, clinical staff, business office, and technical staff);

3. Communication (information materials, test results, and other issues);

4. Physician performance (exam room encounter); and

5. Facility (comfort, cleanliness, parking, and signage).

Following the specific, visit-related issues are four general questions that compose a kind of final report card:

1. Overall satisfaction with the practice;

2. Overall satisfaction with the quality of medical care;

3. Overall satisfaction with one's personal physician or nurse;

4. Willingness to recommend the practice to family members and friends.

The survey fits on two sides of a single sheet of paper, which can increase the response rate without producing survey fatigue (the tendency of respondents to quit part way because they're tired of answering the questions).

The form is anonymous and confidential, although many patients will add their name and phone number, particularly if they want to be contacted to discuss an issue of importance to them.

The rating scale is called a five-point Likert scale. The descriptors conform to the layout of many health plan surveys, with choices ranging from "excellent" to "poor."

Survey Distribution Methods

The practice can distribute the survey either in the office or by mail. Office distribution involves receptionists who ask patients to complete the survey either before leaving the office (depositing the survey in a collection box for anonymity) or when they return home (using a postage-paid reply envelope).

Typical response rates are between 30 to 40 percent, although some practices do better; the difference depends on how the receptionist offers the survey and emphasizes its importance to the practice's efforts to meet patients' expectations for comfortable, hassle-free services.

Mail distribution requires an accurate data file of patient names and addresses. Response rates are typically lower than for in-office surveys (20 to 25 percent, with some exceptions) and the collection period tends to be longer, typically five to six weeks.

Many physicians prefer mail surveys for the protection they offer against manipulation by practice insiders, especially when incentive bonuses depend on the scores. At the same time, mail surveys are about 70 percent more expensive, owing to the costs of list management, mailing services, and outbound and reply postage.

What's Not Good About Telephone Surveys

Telephone surveys can present several issues. First, telephone surveys can often be the most expensive method, but proponents claim a better response rate (some say as high as 85 percent) and that interviewers can probe beyond the basic responses for more detailed and reliable information.

In fact, the reverse is true for several reasons:

- Phone interviews require four to five computerized "dial attempts" to complete a single interview; using this ratio of attempts to completions, the response rate for phone surveys is well below that of office or mail distribution;

- Phone interviews can produce *acquiescence bias* – the tendency of respondents to give socially acceptable answers regardless of the content of the question (often to please the interviewer);

- Because of the relatively rapid question/answer interaction, patients are more likely to give similar answers to a series of questions (*central tendency*), resulting in less variation and less discrimination between survey issues;

- Because respondents are unable to visualize the rating scales, their focus is split between answering the questions and remembering the range of possible choices;

- The negative tone of interviewers probing for dissatisfaction can produce a more negative set of responses; and

- Consumers are often antagonized by attempts to reach them during dinnertime or evening hours (the best time to find patients at home).

The anonymity afforded by self-administered paper surveys and the ability of respondents to answer at their own pace make written-response surveys more likely to produce data you can use. Further, anonymity encourages responses on sensitive issues and intimate details that many respondents are reluctant to discuss with telephone interviewers.

Sample Size and Validity

Surveying every patient in a practice's database would be prohibitively expensive. The population is too large to attempt to survey all of the patients. A small but carefully chosen sample can be used to represent all the patients who come to the practice for their medical care. The sample needs to reflect the characteristics of the population from which it is drawn.

Valid information can be derived from a portion of a practice's entire patient population as long as the sample chosen is representative – that is, the answers from the sample will be as close as possible to what all the patients would say, if they could be asked.

However, sampling has rules. In satisfaction research, the question is, to what extent can the sample in the report be projected across a physician's entire patient population? This question is often unanswerable because everything about every variable in the total population can't be known – age, gender, and so on.

That's why "there is no such thing as a representative, unbiased, fair, or otherwise acceptable sample."[37] A key to valid sampling is to select a random number of patients for the survey. "Random" implies that every person in a practice's patient population has an equal chance of being selected for the survey. In a mailed survey, a random sample can be approximated by asking the computer to select every third patient, or every patient seen on Monday, or by several other criteria. For in-office distribution, a practice can come close to a random sample by choosing a starting point from which every patient is offered a chance to take the survey, until all surveys have been distributed. The assumption is that patients randomize themselves by making an appointment with the doctor during the distribution period.

Assuming the sample is as "random" as it can be made, the next question is, how many surveys are needed to make reasonable statements about how a physician is viewed by his or her patients? A sample size generally agreed on among statisticians (and medical directors) is 30 qualified responses.

The "30 or more" criterion is also nonscientific. It represents a compromise between the money a practice can afford to spend and the statistical validity that will persuade colleagues to accept the results of sampling only a portion of the patient base.

Sample size computations measure only statistical sampling errors; many other sources of error can influence the accuracy and reliability of the survey findings – coverage errors, nonresponse errors, respondent mistakes, questionnaire defects, and administrative

EXHIBIT 7.
Sampling Error for Patient Surveys[38]

Sample Size	Sampling Error (±)
25	16.0%
50	11.2%
75	9.1%
100	7.8%
150	6.4%
250	5.0%
500	3.5%
750	2.9%
1,000	2.5%
1,500	2.0%

errors. Exhibit 7 shows that the sampling error associated with a population of 30 completed surveys is about ±14.0 percent.

There are no guarantees regarding how many patients will complete the survey. Because over-the-counter surveys usually produce response rates of 30 to 40 percent, a distribution of 100 surveys per physician is recommended. If the practice is looking for a summary report for a practice site, a return of 200 completed surveys would have a sampling error of about ±6.0 percent – which, for a marketing study, is sufficient for identifying where the site excels and where it needs to improve.

But what if a physician receives fewer than 30 responses? Can something relevant still be said about the doctor's performance if the sample size is, say, 20 surveys? Sure it can – just not with the same confidence as if the sample size were larger. Conclusions drawn from 20 surveys are valid – just not as valid as conclusions drawn from a larger sample. (These are rough rule-of-thumb numbers – the actual formula for determining sampling error is complex and involves several independent variables.)

A final thought about sample sizes: Because there's no way to eliminate sampling errors completely, what matters most is that all physicians are treated the same – that is, everyone uses the same survey form, the survey is conducted during the same period, and it has the same distribution methodology. If any error in the process is constant across the entire physician population or across all the practices in the benchmarking database, the comparisons are valid even if the scores are less than exact.

◢ Reporting

Survey reports should be designed with the user's needs in mind; the key is to ask, at the start of the project, what does the practice intend to do with the data it receives? Although there are many interesting conclusions that can be drawn from analyzing the data, the primary purposes of the report are to enable practice leaders (1) to identify "what works and what doesn't" in terms of meeting or exceeding patients' expectations for service, and (2) to set priorities for improvement.

The percentage response to each survey question reveals the following:

- "Excellent" and "Very Good" responses represent friends and fans. These respondents are loyal to the practice and would probably resist a competitor's moves to take them away. Their satisfaction also means that they're saying good things about the practice to their families and friends. (Some practices favor using only the "Excellent" percentages like Disney does, believing that anything lower signifies less-than-loyal patients.)

- "Fair" and "Poor" responses signify the opposite. These patients are not loyal and would probably change to another doctor or practice if they suspect that they might receive better service elsewhere. Their dissatisfaction means that they're not saying good things about the practice. (A study by Humana in the 1980s indicated that satisfied patients are likely to tell 2 to 3 others about a particular practice, whereas dissatisfied patients will probably tell 11 to 13 others why they don't like the practice. Other studies put the negative potential even higher. Expressed in marketing terms, the upside potential of satisfying a practice's patients is far outweighed by the downside potential of antagonizing them.)

- The least confidence comes from the "Good" responses. As the midpoint of the scale, the "Good" category can be seen as representing patients who are essentially neutral about the practice. ("Nothing happened that delighted me, but you didn't antagonize me, either.") These patients are like the "undecideds" in an election year – they can stay with the practice or leave, depending on a wide variety of factors.

The bottom line is that the total of "Excellent" and "Very Good" responses indicates a practice's marketing strength; to approximate a practice's potential for losing patients, the percentages in the "Good to Poor" columns can be added.

◢ Other Assessment Strategies

The advantage of setting quantified goals is obvious. Instead of exhorting people to "run faster and work harder," a practice can set a clear target that the nurses and medical assistants can accept, and everyone will know when they reach it. People are more willing to follow a practice's lead if they have a definite goal to shoot for. What's more, it gives the practice a reason to celebrate when they hit the target.

A patient survey is a practice's most valuable measurement tool, but it's not the only way to obtain useful information about the practice's service strengths and weaknesses. Two additional ways are mystery patient assessments and key-person interviews.

Mystery Patient Assessment

Although patient surveys have the advantage of allowing a practice to solicit opinions among large groups of patients, they also have the disadvantage that the questioning is not very deep. Patients circle answers on the rating scale, but their response doesn't tell anything about the specifics behind the scores.

The tool for digging deeper into the strengths and limitations of the practice is the mystery patient assessment. A professional "shopper" – often a person with direct experience working in a medical group – calls for an appointment, goes through the entire encounter, and sends a full report of the experience.

Mystery patients tell you where the practice shines and where it needs polishing. The report exposes exactly what happens during a normal patient encounter and pinpoints the reasons behind the survey scores. The recommendations help the practice make specific changes to the work processes and physician/staff performance that increase patient satisfaction.

Typically, mystery patient reports are confidential. They are sent or presented in person to the practice manager, who decides how the results will be shared with physicians, supervisors, and staff members. (As might be expected, specific comments in the report can arouse defensiveness on the part of the "shopped" physicians and staff if they are broadcast to everyone in the practice.) The report will include the positive aspects of the visit, not just the areas that need improvement. Issues affecting physicians can be reviewed with the president or medical director, who decides what action to take. Issues affecting employees would be shared with appropriate supervisors.

A practice also wants the entire team to know how they're doing as a group. At intervals, a summary report of all mystery patient assessments can be produced. Names and departments can be edited out to avoid shining a negative spotlight on individuals; after all, the assessment is about the entire practice as a team. If it's true that "we're all in this together," then it doesn't matter which person or department the report is about.

As one administrator put it: "If someone praises you, I get to walk in your sunshine; if someone criticizes me, you'll all be tarred with the brush."

Another benefit of mystery patient assessments is this: Whereas a patient survey usually is conducted once or twice each year, during which time physicians and employees can "polish their act," an assessment can occur at any time. Nobody knows when or where the mystery patient will visit, which keeps everyone's attention on service all year round!

Key-Person Interviews

A practice's own people are also a source of valuable assessment information; they see what happens on a daily basis, and often have the best ideas about potential solutions.

Talking with key people in the practice brings them into the practice's strategies for improvement. People who are asked for their input are more likely to support an action plan than those who feel excluded from the assessment process.

Both of these issues can be addressed by adding a schedule of key-person interviews to the preparation for a customer service initiative. Partner physicians, supervisors, and employees can all give an insider's perspective on the challenges they face every day and their insights regarding things to improve. Insiders can report on "what works and what doesn't." Supervisors can provide detailed feedback on performance areas where employees do well and where they don't. Frontline and support staff can add their perspective on teamwork and the working conditions that affect their ability to meet or exceed patient expectations.

Key-person interviews can be one on one or in focus groups. You can review the findings of the patient survey and mystery patient assessments and ask colleagues to comment on the issues raised. A workable interview checklist might contain the following questions:

1. What do you think patients like best and least about our practice?

2. Where do you think we excel at meeting patients' service expectations? Where do we fall short?

3. What's your biggest challenge when you're trying to deliver top-level service to our patients?

4. What usually happens when you hear about a patient who is unhappy with our practice? How do you feel we perform when things go wrong?

5. If you could make one change to improve patient satisfaction, what would it be?

◼ Assessment Report

Now it's time to assemble a report that will be the basis for setting priorities and building a customer service plan. With the patient survey, mystery patient assessments, and key-person interviews to work from, it's time to designate the people who will be responsible for integrating all the input into a single report.

This group of people can be called the Customer Service Committee, and the practice administrator can be in charge of nominating the people who will serve on it.

In a small practice, the administrator might want everyone to be on the committee. For larger practices, a committee that represents a cross section of the practice – physicians, someone from the administrative team, supervisors of key areas, and one or two staff members with seniority and a reputation for participating constructively in meetings – might be considered.

Forming a Customer Service Committee has its own potential pitfall: If the committee members lack sufficient "rank" in the practice, they'll have difficulty getting the attention of senior leadership for their conclusions and recommendations. More than a few customer service initiatives have lost their momentum because responsibility was delegated to people who, although committed, were unable to gain the attention of the practice leadership team.

Chapter 7   Implementing a Plan to Control Pharmaceutical Supplies

SUPPLIES AND EQUIPMENT are the tools that physicians and staff need to function and provide the services that are expected of them. Supplies and equipment include waiting-room chairs and copy paper; consumables, such as scanners, vaccines, and radiology systems; and computers and sophisticated, expensive medical equipment.

These purchases are normally divided into three basic groups: fixed assets, nonbillable supplies, and billable supplies. Fixed assets comprise equipment and instruments that can be used on multiple occasions. They appear on the balance sheet of the practice as an asset and are expensed through the application of depreciation. Nonbillable supplies are those consumables that are used as part of normal everyday operations. The costs of these items cannot be billed to the patient, but they are sometimes billed to specific departments within a practice when detailed cost accounting is desired. Examples of these consumables are pens, paper, alcohol swabs, and syringes.

The last major grouping comprises billable supplies. These are consumable items for which the cost can be passed on to either the patient and/or the third-party payer. The types of supplies included in this category vary based on the specialty of the physician and the rules and regulations that may exist for the state in which the practice is located. Some examples of these billable supplies and the type of practice most likely to stock them are skin care products in dermatology, braces and splints in orthopedics, vaccines in pediatrics and internal medicine, and nutritional supplements in obstetrics. In some cases, the costs of these consumables are not covered by the third-party payer and become the responsibility of the patient. An example of this would be a waterproof casting material instead of standard plaster if a parent whose child has broken an arm or leg wishes the physician to use such an option. The additional cost of this material is normally not covered by the third-party payer, and the patient or guarantor is responsible for the additional cost.

◾ Inventory Control

Unless properly controlled, the purchase, storage, and usage of both billable and nonbillable supplies can become a significant drain on the financial status of the practice. Therefore, guidelines and operating procedures for the ordering, use, and monitoring of supplies should be initiated and maintained. Some examples of these guidelines and procedures are:

- Determination of a schedule for ordering specific groupings of supplies (e.g., clinical, office, pharmaceutical);

- Use of standardized order forms that spell out the specific items that may be ordered;

- Determination of minimum and maximum reorder points to ensure that the organization neither runs out of critical supplies nor stockpiles supplies in quantities that would be categorized as wasteful (these reorder points should be set so that inventory turns over or is completely replaced eight to ten times per year); and

- Periodic checking of the purchase of billable supplies against the amounts that are actually billed to patients. The amounts billed to patients when added to the inventory on hand should equal the amount purchased by the practice. If the amount purchased is higher than the total of the amount billed plus inventory, then the reasons for the inventory shrinkage should be investigated and corrected.

Consumables

The larger the organization, the greater the importance of developing and implementing standards for the various consumable products to ensure that the practice does not begin to maintain stocks of multiple brands of the same product based on the desires of individual members of the organization. By standardizing the consumable products purchased and maintaining specific minimum and maximum reorder points, a practice can maximize savings and reduce costs. Other steps that can be taken to reduce the expenses incurred for consumables include periodically checking prices among various suppliers to ensure the best price and negotiating longer-term contracts whereby the practice is committing to purchase specified products from a supplier for fixed prices.

Equipment and Supplies

When purchasing equipment, other issues should be addressed to ensure that the practice receives the greatest value for the dollar expended. Whether for meeting clinical or administrative demands, the purchaser needs to evaluate the different models and types of equipment available on the market. In addition to evaluating whether the equipment will meet the operational needs of the organization, the costs of the equipment, including acquisition costs (whether purchase or lease), cost of supplies needed to maintain the equipment, maintenance contracts, and any construction renovations needed to maintain and operate the equipment should be assessed. Once the final decision is made on the specific make and model of equipment to be purchased, it is the responsibility of the designated administrative officer to not only negotiate the best offer for the equipment but to periodically evaluate the equipment to ensure that it continues to meet the organization's needs in an efficient and cost-effective manner.

In addition, the purchaser should consider that the utilization of these supplies will result in the creation of various waste products that must be disposed of in a proper and timely manner.

Arrangements should be made to properly dispose of biohazardous waste products, including syringes, sharps (e.g., needles and scalpels), and any products that have been contaminated with bodily fluids and blood. Failure to properly dispose of these items can result in an exposure risk to other patients and staff. Normally, this type of disposal is handled through contracts with licensed companies.

A second significant waste product issue involves the disposal of documentation that may contain a patient's name and other private information. These waste documents may include daily appointment schedules and duplicate telephone messages. To ensure compliance with the Health Insurance Portability and Accountability Act guidelines, all of these documents should be properly shredded, which involves either obtaining the equipment necessary to internally shred the documents in question or contracting with an independent, bonded shredding company to perform this task and provide receptacles to secure the documents until they are properly destroyed.

Pharmaceuticals

A final category of supplies, which touches upon all of the previous areas of discussion and has several additional issues, is pharmaceuticals. Within a practice, this category may have several distinct subgroupings, based on the practice's specialty. These subgroupings may include vaccines, injectible medications (e.g., Solu-Medrol, Depo-Medrol, vitamin B-12), narcotics, and samples of prescription medications. With the exception of samples, all of these items would be considered billable consumable supplies.

The maintenance of pharmaceutical supplies within a practice is subject to various federal, state, and local regulations and laws. Narcotics and other controlled substances must be kept in secured locations (e.g., double-locked safes or metal boxes) that are not accessible to unauthorized staff or others. In addition, logs must be kept of the utilization of these drugs, and periodic confirmatory inventories must be accomplished. The logs for each pharmaceutical should document the final disposition of all narcotics and controlled substances purchased or received by the practice. All of these documents must be available to designated government investigators charged with the responsibility to ensure compliance with regulatory safeguards.

The practice needs to ensure that all other pharmaceuticals are appropriately secured and dispensed in a clinically correct and safe manner. Because many pharmaceuticals and vaccines have significant costs and short shelf lives, the practice should implement and maintain strong inventory systems, including rotation of stock to ensure that inventory does not reach its expiration date, tracking of utilization to ensure that all usage has been properly billed, and proper disposal of out-of-date items. Many out-of-date pharmaceuticals can be returned to the manufacturer or supplier for credit toward new inventory. Additionally, this inventory should be kept in centralized locked cabinets to ensure that they will be properly maintained and distributed.

Samples

The use of pharmaceutical samples within practices has become a significant issue of control, storage, and maintenance. The practice may be inundated with pharmaceutical sales representatives whose function is to provide information on why their particular pharmaceutical is the best as well as to provide the practice with samples for patient use. The practice needs to set inventory controls in place when accepting these samples, or the practice may find itself with significant excess quantities of a specific drug. Once the practice has accepted these samples for distribution to patients, it has also accepted responsibility for the proper storage, control, and the ultimate disposal of these samples. The same inventory problems and issues that are addressed with pharmaceuticals that are purchased by the practice also should apply to these pharmaceutical samples. Most practices secure the samples in cabinets or closets that are locked when the practice is closed. Because of the volume involved, a major issue for a practice is the disposal of samples that have passed their expiration date. These samples cannot be returned to the manufacturer, and the responsibility falls on the practice to properly dispose of them. This disposal process can become extremely time-consuming and expensive for the practice.

Summary

All of these items directly affect the bottom line of the organization. As such, it is important for the medical practice executive to monitor these costs and track them within the appropriate department or cost center.

Conclusion

THIS VOLUME has touched on the skill sets needed to become adept in accomplishing the tasks within the Patient Care Systems domain within the *Medical Practice Management Body of Knowledge (BOK), second edition*. The information provided should assist the medical practice administrator in addressing and responding to the ongoing clinical demands of his or her practice.

It is important to remember that to maximize the effectiveness of these skill sets, they should be kept within the context and understanding of the basic principles of four general competencies:

1. Professionalism;

2. Leadership;

3. Communication skills; and

4. Critical thinking skills.

Without the knowledge that can be obtained from a full understanding of all competencies within the BOK, it will be difficult to properly apply the knowledge that is obtained from any one competency or skill.

Exercises

THESE QUESTIONS have been retired from the ACMPE Essay Exam question bank. Because there are so many ways to handle various situations, there are no "right" answers, and thus, no answer key. Use these questions to help you practice responses in different scenarios.

1. You are the administrator of a busy 12-provider orthopedic practice. Your medical group is well established within your community, and over the past several years it has experienced strong referral patterns from most of the community's primary care practices. One of your senior surgeons has come to you with concerns that he has noticed a decrease in referrals from two primary care practices. He tells you he thinks several of the former primary care physicians retired, and he has noticed that the new physicians do not seem to be referring as many patients to him. He has asked you for specific recommendations to address the problem.

   Describe how you would handle this situation.

2. You are the administrator of a 35-physician multispecialty group in a metropolitan area. During the past year, patient visits have decreased by 20 percent. Several members of the executive committee believe that there has been a shift in market share to other new physicians who have moved to the community. Other board members believe that the shift has been a result of poor patient service. The board has asked you to develop a specific plan of action to reverse this trend.

    Describe how you would handle this situation.

3. You are the administrator for a primary care medical practice serving a growing suburban community. It is becoming increasingly difficult to schedule patient appointments, and waiting times are increasing. The physicians disagree about the need to recruit new providers.

   Describe how you would handle this situation.

4. You are an administrator of a medical group practice. A patient presents to the clinic and states that she has an appointment. The receptionist checks the schedule and does not find an appointment for this patient. The patient insists she was given the appointment time and has a reminder card at home to prove she is accurate. The receptionist states that the doctor already has a full schedule for the morning. The patient is upset and demands to be seen.

Describe how would you handle this situation.

5. You are the administrator of a 40-physician multispecialty
    medical group with several locations. Each clinic is responsi-
    ble for ordering, maintaining, and distributing patient care
    supplies, including pharmaceuticals. Each of these locations
    also has extensive supplies of sample medications. Your
    new director of nursing has reported missing pharmaceu-
    ticals and sample medications from at least two different
    locations during the past week. Her initial investigation
    reveals that there are no written policies or formal inven-
    tory control processes in place.

    What course of action would you take in this situation?

Notes

1. Reprinted from *MGMA Connexion*, January 2008, with permission from the Medical Group Management Association.

2. I. S. Kirsh, A. Jungeblut, L. Jenkins, and A. Kolstad. Adult Literacy in America: A First Look at the Findings of the National Adult Literacy Survey (Washington, DC: National Center for Education Statistics, August 1993), http://nces.ed.gov/naal/index.asp?file=OtherResources/ExecSumAdultL-itFirstLook.asp&PageId=156 (accessed May 29, 2007).

3. Ibid.

4. B. D. Weiss, *20 Common Problems in Primary Care* (New York: McGraw-Hill, December 1999).

5. Ibid.

6. Ibid.

7. D. W. Baker, J. A. Gazmararian, M. V. Williams, T. Scott, R. M. Parker, D. Green, et al., "Functional Health Literacy and the Risk of Hospital Admission Among Medicare Managed Care Enrollees," *American Journal of Public Health* 92 (2002): 1278–1283.

8. Kirsh et al.

9. Weiss.

10. Kirsh et al.

11. Ibid.

12. Ibid.

13. This chapter is reprinted from *Rx for Business Success: Joining a Medical Practice*, copyright 2005, with permission of Medical Group Management Association. All rights reserved.

14. Stephanie J. Lee, Anthony L. Back, Susan D. Block, and Susan K. Stewart, "Enhancing Physician-Patient Communication," in *Hematology: American Society of Hematology Education Program*, 464–483, www.entrepreneur. com/article/0,4621,310647,00.html (accessed Sept. 17, 2005).

15. Office for the Advancement of Telehealth, "Welcome Page," telehealth. hrsa.gov/welcome.htm (accessed Oct. 18, 2005).

16. Ibid.

17. M. Tervalon and J. Murray-Garcia, "Cultural Humility vs. Cultural Competence: A Critical Distinction in Defining Physician Training Outcomes in Medical Education," *Journal of Health Care Poor Underserved* 9 (1998): 117–125.

18. Ibid.

19. Vincent T. Covello and Miley W. Merkhofer, *Risk Assessment Methods: Approaches for Assessing Health and Environmental Risks* (New York: Plenum Press, 1993).

20. New York State Department of Health, New York State Community Health Assessment (CHA) Guidance Documents, www.health.state.ny.us/nysdoh/chac (accessed Oct. 19, 2005).

21. Ibid.

22. Ibid.

23. Ibid.

24. U.S. Department of Health and Human Services, *Healthy People 2010*, 2nd edition, With *Understanding and Improving Health*, and *Objectives for Improving Health*. 2 Vols. (Washington, DC: U.S. Government Printing Office, November 2000).

25. Al Lautenslager, 2003, "PR Is More Than Just Press Releases," www.entrepreneur.com/article/0,4621,310647,00.html (accessed Oct. 19, 2005).

26. Ibid.

27. National Association of City and County Health Officials (NACCHO), "NACCHO Public Health Communications Toolkit," http://archive.naccho.org/documents/Communication-toolkit.pdf (accessed Sept. 18, 2005).

28. Ibid.

29. Ibid.

30. Adapted and reprinted with permission from *A+ Marketing: Proven Tactics for Success*, published by Medical Group Management Association.

31. Brian Mathwich, "Using the Process Map to Improve Your Bottom Line," *MGMA Connexion* 4, no. 6 (2004): 31.

32. Elizabeth Woodcock, *Mastering Patient Flow* (Englewood, CO: Medical Group Management Association, 2003), 88.

33. Austin Ross, Stephen J. Williams, and Ernest J. Pavlock, *Ambulatory Care Management* (Englewood, CO: Medical Group Management Association, 1998), 196.

34. This chapter is reprinted from *Rx for Business Success: Joining a Medical Practice*, copyright 2005, with permission of Medical Group Management Association. All rights reserved.

35. This chapter is reprinted from Kevin W. Sullivan, *Star-Studded Service: Six Steps to Winning Patient Satisfaction*, copyright 2007, with permission from Medical Group Management Association. All rights reserved.

36. The MGMA-Sullivan/Luallin Patient Survey Program[SM] maintains the largest current-year ambulatory database in health care. The national database is built from more than 400 patient surveys each year and contains more than 300,000 individual patient responses. For a copy of the survey form, or more information on calculating beta coefficient using stepwise regression, contact the authors at inquiry@sullivan-luallin.com.

37. Stuart 1968, as cited in Kevin W. Sullivan, *Star-Studded Service: Six Steps to Winning Patient Satisfaction* (Englewood, CO: Medical Group Management Association, 2007).

38. J. L. Weeks et al., 1996, as cited in Kevin W. Sullivan, *Star-Studded Service: Six Steps to Winning Patient Satisfaction* (Englewood, CO: Medical Group Management Association, 2007).

Bibliography

Eliscu, A. T., *Ready-Set-Market!* (Englewood, CO: Medical Group Management Association, 1999).

Peppers, D., and M. Rogers, *The One to One Future: Building Relationships One Customer at a Time* (New York: Doubleday and Company, 1996).

Index

Note: (ex.) indicates exhibit.